Living Boldly with Endo

The Essential Guide to Coping and Thriving Despite Endometriosis

Theodora Bagwell

Copyright@ 2024

Table of Contents

Preface

Millions of people worldwide suffer from endometriosis, however the condition is frequently misdiagnosed and misunderstood. The purpose of this guide is to help people coping with the difficulties associated with this condition by offering clear, helpful information.

I have personally experienced the anguish, perplexity, and frustration that many people with endometriosis go through. I created this book to provide a thorough resource for comprehending symptoms, looking into possible treatments, and coming up with ideas to make life better on a daily basis.

Understanding the causes, risk factors, and treatment of endometriosis is provided in each chapter, along with advice tailored specifically for adolescent and postmenopausal women. It is my desire that this book gives you the confidence to take charge of your health, get the care you require, and realize that you are not alone.

With empathy and support,
Theodora Bagwell

Chapter One

Understanding Endometriosis

Endometriosis is more than just a medical condition; it's a deeply personal and often misunderstood experience that affects millions of women worldwide.

How it manifests, and why it can have such a profound impact on the lives of those who live with it. When endometrial, or tissue resembling the uterine lining, starts to proliferate outside the uterus, endometriosis develops.

This tissue is present in the pelvic cavity as well as on the uterus' exterior, the fallopian tubes, and the ovaries. Rarely, it could extend past the pelvic organs.

This tissue thickens, degrades, and bleeds as it usually would throughout the menstrual cycle every month.

This misplaced tissue, however, is unable to depart the body, in contrast to the uterine lining, which does so during menstruation. This results in pain, inflammation, and the development of adhesions, or scar tissue.

The Prevalence of Endometriosis

Endometriosis is a prevalent ailment that impacts roughly 10% of women who are able to procreate. It is still frequently misdiagnosed and misinterpreted while being very common.

Before receiving a proper diagnosis, many women endure years of suffering in secret, frequently being assured that their agony is "normal" or "in their heads."

Being aware of endometriosis and its effects on an individual's physical, mental, and social well-being is the first step towards comprehending the condition.

Symptoms of Endometriosis

The symptoms of endometriosis can take many different forms, and each person may experience the disease to varying degrees of severity. Typical symptoms include:

- Pelvic Pain
- Painful Periods (Dysmenorrhea)
- Pain During Intercourse
- Pain with Bowel Movements or Urination
- Excessive Bleeding
- Infertility

It's crucial to remember that the degree of the ailment is not always correlated with how bad the pain is.

While some women with advanced endometriosis may have little to no discomfort, others with moderate endometriosis may feel considerable pain.

Endometriosis is a disorder that can impact a woman's entire life; it is not merely a physical one. Emotional anguish, anxiety, and depression can result from the chronic pain and its associated symptoms.

There may be a significant negative effect on relationships, employment, and day-to-day activities, which can leave one feeling powerless and alone.

Many endometriosis sufferers claim that friends, family, and even medical professionals misunderstand them. This lack of knowledge and assistance can make dealing with a chronic illness more emotionally taxing.

Diagnosis

The challenge of receiving a diagnosis is one of the most annoying features of endometriosis. Women typically have to wait seven to ten years following the onset of symptoms before receiving a proper diagnosis. A number of reasons, such as the normalization of menstrual pain, health care practitioners' lack of understanding, and the limitations of available diagnostic instruments, frequently contribute to this delay.

Laparoscopy, a minimally invasive surgical procedure that enables doctors to inspect the inside of the abdomen and obtain samples of any questionable tissue, is the gold standard for detecting endometriosis.

Even with this method, diagnosis remains difficult, and many women receive incorrect diagnoses before learning the true diagnosis.

Chapter Two

The Medical Perspective

Anyone dealing with endometriosis must comprehend the medical aspects of the disorder. The science of endometriosis, including an examination of its effects on the body, potential treatments, and the difficulties in treating it medically.

A disorder with deep roots in the intricate mechanisms of the human body is endometriosis. It is the development of tissue that resembles endometrial tissue outside the uterus, where it shouldn't be.

With each menstrual cycle, this rogue tissue undergoes the same changes as the tissue inside the uterus, including thickening, breaking down, and bleeding.

Nevertheless, this exterior tissue cannot leave the body, in contrast to the tissue inside the uterus, which does so after menstruation. Inflammation, the development of scar tissue (adhesions), and cysts—particularly endometriomas—occur as a result.

Numerous issues may arise as a result of this aberrant tissue growth. Adhesions can cause organs to stay together, which can seriously impair the reproductive, digestive, and urinary systems.

Inflammation can also cause excruciating pain. Ovulation and fertility may also be hampered by ovarian cyst development.

Stages of Endometriosis

Based on the amount, position, and depth of the endometrial implants, as well as the existence and severity of adhesions and ovarian cysts, endometriosis is categorized into four stages:

Stage 1 (Minimal): Small, superficial implants and possibly minor adhesions.

Stage 2 (Mild): More implants, both superficial and deeper, as well as more adhesions.

Stage 3 (Moderate): Numerous deep implants, small cysts on one or both ovaries, and more significant adhesions.

Stage 4 (Severe): Many deep implants, large cysts on one or both ovaries, and extensive adhesions.

It's crucial to understand that the severity of symptoms is not always correlated with the stage of endometriosis. While a woman with stage 4 endometriosis may have little to no discomfort, a woman with stage 1 endometriosis may feel excruciating pain.

Treatment Options

Treatment for endometriosis frequently entails a mix of strategies based on the symptoms, objectives, and general health of the patient. The following are the main medical interventions now in use:

Hormonal Therapies: By reducing or eliminating menstruation, hormone therapy may help halt or limit the formation of endometrial tissue. Among these therapies are:

Birth Control Pills: By delaying the menstrual cycle, oral contraceptives are frequently the first line of treatment and can significantly lessen or eliminate pain.

Gonadotropin-Releasing Hormone (GnRH) Agonists: These medications cause the endometrial tissue to shrink and estrogen levels to drop temporarily, akin to a menopause.

Progestins: Progestin therapy can help suppress menstruation and relieve symptoms. It can be administered as tablets, injections, or IUDs.

Aromatase Inhibitors: These medications lower the production of estrogen and are occasionally used in conjunction with other hormonal therapies.

Handling Pain: One of the most crippling effects of endometriosis is pain. Multifaceted approaches are often necessary for effective pain management:

NSAIDs: Ibuprofen and other non-steroidal anti-inflammatory medications are frequently used to treat pain and inflammation.

Nerve Blockers: In rare circumstances, injections to block nerves can relieve excruciating pelvic discomfort.

Opioids: In severe cases, Opioids may be administered for short-term pain relief, but they are generally not advised for long-term usage due to the danger of dependence.

Surgical Interventions: When endometriosis affects fertility or the symptoms are severe, surgery is frequently required. The primary surgical alternatives consist of:

Laparoscopy: The most popular surgical procedure for treating endometriosis, laparoscopy is a minimally invasive technique that can be used to remove or eliminate adhesions, cysts, and endometrial implants.

Laparotomy: When all other therapies have failed, a laparotomy—a more intrusive surgery than a laparoscopy—may be used to treat severe endometriosis.

Hysterectomy: In severe situations, a hysterectomy (removal of the uterus) may be considered, especially if previous therapies have failed and the patient has no intention of becoming pregnant. Usually a last option, this procedure may or may not involve ovarian excision (oophorectomy).

The Role of the Immune System

According to research, endometriosis may be significantly influenced by the immune system during its onset and course. The immune system does not seem to be able to identify and get rid of the displaced endometrial tissue in women who have endometriosis.

When it comes to endometriosis, early intervention can greatly enhance results. Early diagnosis and treatment of endometriosis can lower the risk of complications, stop the disease from getting worse, and enhance the quality of life for those who have it.

However, many women do not acquire an early diagnosis because the symptoms are frequently ambiguous and variable.

Treatment Options Complexities

Selecting a course of treatment for endometriosis is not always simple. It entails assessing the advantages and disadvantages of each choice while taking the patient's symptoms, objectives (such pain management or fertility preservation), and preferences into account.

For some, maintaining fertility may be the main objective, which could explain their desire for less intrusive procedures or particular kinds of surgery.

Others may prioritize lessening discomfort and enhancing day-to-day functioning, which may result in other therapeutic options.

The complexity of treatment choices emphasizes the value of individualized care and the necessity for patients and health care providers to collaborate closely to create a plan that is tailored to each patient's particular requirements and situation.

Chapter Three

Living with Endometriosis

Endometriosis-related living is a difficult path with many special difficulties, emotional highs and lows, and a need for continuous adaptation.

Despite the difficulties endometriosis may cause, you can have a happy life by learning about your body, properly managing your symptoms, and getting the assistance you need.

Understanding Your Body and Symptoms

Since endometriosis affects people differently, it's important to know how your body presents with the disease. The range of symptoms is broad and includes everything from severe menstrual pain to persistent exhaustion, digestive problems, and even infertility. You can better control your symptoms if you are aware of your body's cues.

It can be beneficial to keep a thorough log of your symptoms in order to spot trends and triggers. Jot down any additional symptoms you have, such as bloating or weariness, as well as the time the pain started, how it felt, and what you were doing at the time.

An abrupt worsening of symptoms is called a flare-up. Stress, particular diets, hormone fluctuations, or physical exertion can all cause them. You can better avoid or control your triggers if you are aware of them.

Pain Management Strategies

One prevalent and frequently incapacitating sign of endometriosis is pain. Effective pain management necessitates a multifaceted strategy catered to your individual requirements.

For mild to severe pain, over-the-counter medications like ibuprofen or naproxen may be helpful.

Prescription drugs such hormone therapies or muscle relaxants could be required for more severe pain. Be sure to speak with your doctor before beginning any new drug.

Menstrual cramps and pelvic pain can be instantly relieved by applying a heating pad or hot water bottle to your lower back or abdomen.

Pain in the pelvis can be reduced and muscular function can be enhanced with specialized pelvic floor physical therapy. You can follow exercises and stretches prescribed by a physical therapist.

Nutrition and Lifestyle Changes

Managing the symptoms of endometriosis can be greatly impacted by adopting a healthy lifestyle. Although there isn't a particular diet for endometriosis, there are several foods that can help lower inflammation and enhance general health.

Eat a diet rich in whole grains, fruits, vegetables, and omega-3 fatty acids, which are foods that reduce inflammation. Limiting red meat, sugar, and processed food intake can also aid in the management of inflammation.

Water consumption is important for general health and can aid with digestion and bloating management.

Frequent, mild exercise helps elevate mood and lessen discomfort. Physical activities such as yoga, swimming, and walking are easy on the body and have many advantages.

Chapter Four

Fertility and Endometriosis

Concerns around fertility and the possibility of conception can be a major source of stress and anxiety for a large number of individuals with endometriosis.

Although endometriosis is known to impact fertility in a variety of ways, being aware of the illness and your alternatives can enable you to make well-informed decisions regarding your reproductive health.

Depending on the degree and location of endometrial tissue, endometriosis can affect fertility in a number of ways:

Anatomical Deformities: Adhesions and cysts, two conditions brought on by severe endometriosis, have the potential to change the structure of the reproductive organs. Adhesions, for instance, can clog or twist the fallopian tubes, which makes it harder for the egg to pass from the ovaries into the uterus.

Inflammation: The uterus, fallopian tubes, and ovaries can all be negatively impacted by the inflammation brought on by endometrial implants, which may make it more difficult to fertilize or implant.

Ovulation and Egg Quality: The precise mechanisms in underlying endometriosis impact on these processes remains unclear, but certain studies indicate that it may have an effect on either.

Immune System: Endometriosis may alter the pelvic immunological milieu, creating unfavorable conditions for sperm survival and fertilization.

It's crucial to remember that many endometriosis sufferers are able to conceive, either naturally or with the help of a doctor. Each person's experience with endometriosis and its effect on fertility is unique.

Fertility Options

It's crucial to understand that there are various fertility alternatives accessible if you have endometriosis and are thinking about establishing a family.

The best option for you will depend on your particular circumstances, age, the severity of your endometriosis, and your general health.

Many people with mild to moderate endometriosis are able to become pregnant spontaneously. You might think about trying to conceive naturally if your symptoms are under control and there are no major adhesions or cysts affecting your reproductive tissue.

Depending on your unique situation, your healthcare professional can help you understand your odds of conceiving naturally.

Fertility Treatments

Ovulation Induction: Drugs that cause the ovaries to release eggs are used in this procedure. To improve the odds of pregnancy, it is frequently used in conjunction with timed sex or intrauterine insemination (IUI).

Intrauterine Insemination (IUI): To aid in conception, IUI is injecting sperm directly into the uterus at the approximate time of ovulation. Those with mild to moderate endometriosis may benefit from this approach.

In vitro fertilization (IVF): When other fertility treatments have failed or there is severe endometriosis with notable anatomical deformities, IVF is sometimes regarded as the most effective treatment for endometriosis. During in vitro fertilization (IVF), the ovaries are stimulated to generate several eggs, the eggs are extracted, fertilized in a lab, and the resultant embryos are inserted into the uterus.

Surgery to remove adhesions, cysts, and endometrial lesions may occasionally enhance the success of infertility. The most popular method, laparoscopy surgery, can aid in the restoration of normal anatomy and function.

Depending on your desired level of fertility and the severity of your endometriosis, your doctor will talk to you about whether surgery is a good option for you.

Planning for the Future

There are proactive measures you may take right now if you have endometriosis and are worried about your ability to conceive in the future.

Consider fertility preservation methods like egg or embryo freezing if you're not ready to become pregnant but are worried about your future fertility. These choices can boost your chances of eventually starting a family while also giving you piece of mind.

Consult your gynecologist or fertility specialist on a regular basis to track the development of endometriosis and determine any possible effects on your reproductive system. Making educated decisions regarding your reproductive health can be facilitated by remaining proactive.

Remain up to date with the most recent findings and developments about endometriosis and reproductive therapies. Reproductive medicine is a rapidly developing discipline, with new possibilities and treatments appearing on a regular basis.

Chapter Five

Integrative and Holistic Methods

Treatments for endometriosis are frequently not enough to manage it. A lot of people discover that their overall well-being and symptom management are enhanced when holistic and integrative treatments are included in their treatment plan.

Treating the full person—mind, body, and spirit—rather than merely the disease's symptoms is the goal of holistic and integrated medicine.

Patients can address many facets of their health by combining complementary therapies with traditional medical treatments.

To encourage general health and well being by emphasizing dietary adjustments, stress reduction, and natural remedies that aid in the body's natural healing processes.

Integrating medical and complementary therapies can aid with pain management, stress reduction, mental wellness, and energy restoration.

Diet and Nutrition

Nutrition and diet are very important in the management of endometriosis. Although there isn't a single diet that may treat endometriosis, some dietary adjustments can help lower inflammation and lessen symptoms.

Eating foods that lower bodily inflammation can aid in the management of pain and other symptoms.

Make sure to include lots of nutritious grains, fruits, veggies, and lean proteins. Walnuts, flax seeds, and seafood all contain omega-3 fatty acids, which are particularly healthy.

Certain foods have the potential to worsen endometriosis symptoms. Red meat, dairy, gluten, caffeine, and processed foods are a few examples of them. Maintaining a meal journal might assist in recognizing and avoiding specific trigger foods.

Make sure your diet includes foods like leafy greens, berries, nuts, seeds, and seafood that are high in vitamins and minerals that promote hormone balance and immunological function.

Maintaining adequate hydration is crucial for general health as it can lessen bloating and enhance digestion.

Physical Activity and Exercise

Frequent exercise helps to improve general health and manage the symptoms of endometriosis. Exercise helps control pain, lessen inflammation, and elevate mood.

Exercises that are easy on the body and can help relieve pain and stiffness include walking, swimming, and cycling. Additionally, Pilates and yoga help build muscle, increase flexibility, and encourage calm.

Increasing muscle strength helps ease discomfort and support joints. Emphasize low-impact strength training activities with resistance bands or light weights.

Stress reduction and relaxation are encouraged by the integration of physical movement with mindfulness and breath control found in practices like yoga, tai chi, and qigong.

Alternative Therapies

Additional relief from endometriosis symptoms might be obtained through complementary and alternative therapy.

In addition to medical treatments, these therapies can assist manage pain, lower stress levels, and enhance general well being.

Acupuncture: This traditional Chinese medicine relieves pain and encourages healing by introducing tiny needles into certain body sites. Acupuncture is a popular way for endometriosis sufferers to manage their pelvic discomfort and lower their stress levels.

Herbal Medicine: A number of herbs, including evening primrose oil, turmeric, and ginger, have anti-inflammatory qualities that may help control endometriosis symptoms.

To be sure they are safe and won't conflict with other prescriptions, it is imperative to speak with a healthcare professional before beginning any herbal supplementation.

Massage Therapy: Therapeutic massage therapy is a useful tool for easing pain, promoting better circulation, and reducing muscle tension. Additionally helpful in easing pelvic pain and discomfort are specialized abdominal or pelvic massages.

Chiropractic Care: By enhancing spinal alignment and lowering nerve irritation, chiropractic adjustments may be able to assist some people manage endometriosis-related discomfort.

Stress Reduction Techniques

Endometriosis symptoms can be made worse by prolonged stress, thus managing stress is an essential component of a comprehensive care plan.

Being attentive requires focusing on the here and now without passing judgment. Frequent mindfulness meditation can be beneficial in lowering the levels of stress, anxiety, and sadness that are frequently linked to chronic pain diseases such as endometriosis.

Deep breathing exercises, such box breathing and diaphragmatic breathing, can ease discomfort, lower stress levels, and soothe the neurological system.

To ease physical tension and stress, progressive muscle relaxation, or PMR, entails tensing and then relaxing various muscle groups. It's a straightforward yet powerful method for easing pain and encouraging calm.

Importance of Rest

Getting enough sleep is crucial for general health and well being, especially for people who are coping with a chronic illness like endometriosis.

Make sure your sleeping environment is cozy and restful, set up a regular sleep schedule, and establish a calming nighttime ritual.

Sleep can be disrupted by endometriosis pain and discomfort. To enhance the quality of your sleep, try utilizing body-supporting pillows, a comfy mattress, and relaxation techniques. You can also speak with a health care professional for more recommendations.

To control exhaustion and sustain energy levels, pay attention to your body's needs and take naps or rest periods as necessary.

Mental and Emotional Health Support

Emotional and mental health can suffer from having endometriosis. In order to manage the illness holistically, these factors must be taken into consideration.

Having a conversation with a therapist or counselor can assist in addressing the emotional difficulties brought on by endometriosis, including grief, anxiety, and sadness.

For the treatment of chronic pain, cognitive-behavioral therapy (CBT) and acceptance and commitment therapy (ACT) are especially useful.

Be it online or in person, joining a support group can offer a feeling of community, practical guidance, and emotional support. Having someone who can relate to and validate your experiences can be immensely reassuring and validating.

Processing emotions and managing stress can be therapeutically achieved by writing your thoughts, feelings, and experiences. It can also be used to monitor emotional health symptoms and spot trends.

Chapter Six

Causes and Risk Factors

Millions of individuals worldwide suffer with endometriosis, yet its precise cause is still unknown. There is a strong hereditary component to endometriosis.

You may be more susceptible to endometriosis if your mother, sister, or another close family has it. This clear reminder that endometriosis is inherited rather than "in your head" comes from this family connection.

It is imperative to ascertain one's family medical history as there is evidence indicating that specific genes associated with inflammation and immunological response may predispose an individual to endometriosis. Telling your health care practitioner if endometriosis runs in your family will help to ensure appropriate monitoring and prompt action.

Endometriosis is sometimes referred to be an estrogen-driven disorder, meaning that high estrogen conditions are ideal for the growth of the disease. Among its many other effects, the hormone estrogen promotes the development of endometrial tissue.

This can include the endometrial-like tissue that proliferates outside the uterus in those who have endometriosis. Hormonal imbalances, especially those involving elevated estrogen or decreased progesterone, can provide the ideal environment for the onset and progression of endometriosis.

Nonetheless, the immune system appears to be lacking in its response to endometriosis patients. The immune system permits the endometrial-like tissue to continue developing outside the uterus rather than identifying and eliminating it.

This malfunction may result in long-term inflammation, which exacerbates pain and promotes the growth of scar tissue.

More often than not, we are unaware of the impact that our surroundings have on our health. Endometriosis risk has been associated with exposure to specific chemicals, including PCBs and dioxins.

These substances have the ability to upset the body's delicate hormonal balance, which may lead to the growth of endometrial-like tissue in inappropriate areas.

Even though it is hard to completely avoid environmental toxins, people may advocate for a healthier environment and make educated decisions about their exposure by being aware of these poisons' potential effects.

Retrograde menstruation is one of the most widely recognized ideas for how endometriosis develops. When menstrual blood enters the pelvic cavity through the fallopian tubes in reverse rather than exiting the body, this happens.

Endometrial cells, which have the ability to settle and proliferate in the pelvic region, are present in this blood. Although many people have retrograde menstruation, not everyone goes on to develop endometriosis, indicating that there may be additional factors at work in addition to genetic susceptibility and immune system dysfunction.

There are specific menstrual traits that may indicate an increased risk of endometriosis. The risk of having endometriosis might be raised by variables such early menstrual onset, brief menstrual cycles, heavy menstrual flow, and protracted periods.

These elements are thought to raise the possibility of retrograde menstruation or other processes that promote the growth of tissue outside the uterus that resembles endometrial tissue.

It's important to talk to your health care physician about any menstrual features you may have, particularly if you have symptoms that may indicate endometriosis.

Chapter Seven

Symptoms and Diagnosis

Endometriosis is commonly known as the "invisible illness" because to its highly variable symptoms that are often misinterpreted or disregarded.

Typical Symptoms

Since endometriosis presents differently in every individual, diagnosis can be extremely difficult. Nonetheless, a number of symptoms are frequently connected to the illness:

- Pelvic Pain
- Painful Periods (Dysmenorrhea)
- Chronic Pain
- Pain During Intercourse (Dyspareunia)
- Heavy Menstrual Bleeding (Menorrhagia)
- Gastrointestinal Symptoms

- Urinary Symptoms
- Fatigue Infertility

Adverse Symptoms

Although the preceding symptoms are frequently linked to endometriosis, there are other, less common symptoms that may complicate the diagnosis:

- Chest Aches and Bloody Coughs
- Sciatic Pain
- Neurological Symptoms

There is a high rate of misdiagnosis due to the symptoms of endometriosis being mistaken for ovarian cysts, fibroid, IBS, and pelvic inflammatory disease (PID).

Even in the medical community, endometriosis is still not well understood and under diagnosed despite how common it is.

Diagnosis

Examining the patient's symptoms and medical history in detail is the first step in diagnosing endometriosis. This involves talking about pain thresholds, menstrual cycles, and any endometriosis in the family.

Pelvic exams are useful for detecting anomalies like cysts or scars behind the uterus, but they are not always successful in endometriosis diagnosis, particularly when the lesions are tiny or situated deeper in the pelvic cavity.

To exclude other illnesses or detect endometriosis-related cysts, such endometriomas (often referred to as "chocolate cysts"), ultrasound and magnetic resonance imaging (MRI) are frequently utilized. However, because they do not identify every endometrial lesion, these imaging techniques are unable to provide a conclusive diagnosis of endometriosis.

The laparoscopy, a minimally invasive surgical procedure, is the gold standard for detecting endometriosis. In order to visually inspect for endometrial lesions, a minor incision is made to insert a small camera into the pelvic cavity during this surgery.

In the course of the operation, lesions that are discovered may be excised or biopsied. Although laparoscopy offers a conclusive diagnosis, it is a surgical treatment with risks and recovery time involved.

The gold standard for diagnosing endometriosis is a minimally invasive surgical procedure called laparoscopy. During this procedure, a small camera is inserted into the pelvic cavity through a tiny incision, allowing the surgeon to visually inspect for endometrial lesions.

If lesions are found, they can be biopsied or removed during the same procedure. While laparoscopy provides a definitive diagnosis, it is a surgical procedure and comes with associated risks and recovery time.

Chapter Eight

Surgical Treatment Options

When managing endometriosis, surgery is frequently essential, particularly for those who have not responded to medication or lifestyle modifications. Surgical methods can increase fertility and significantly reduce pain.

Surgery, however, is not a cure, so you should carefully evaluate your options with your health care professional before deciding to have surgery.

When diagnosing and treating endometriosis, surgery can be very important, especially for those who have significant symptoms, a more advanced stage of the disease, or difficulty conceiving.

Endometriosis is a chronic illness, despite the fact that surgery can alleviate pain and enhance reproductive success. Recurrence is a possible even after surgery. As much of the endometrial-like tissue as feasible must be removed or destroyed during surgery in order to relieve discomfort and return the damaged organs to normal function.

Types of Surgical Procedures

There are various surgical techniques for treating endometriosis; each has advantages, disadvantages, and possible results of its own.

The degree of the illness, the patient's symptoms, and their desire for future fertility all influence the surgical option.

Laparoscopy: Laparoscopy is a minimally invasive surgical technique that is the gold standard for endometriosis diagnosis and treatment.

A tiny abdominal incision is made in order to put a tiny camera, known as a laparoscope, into the pelvic cavity during this treatment.

This enables the surgeon to visually examine the pelvic organs for cysts, adhesions, and endometrial abnormalities. If endometrial tissue is discovered, it can be removed surgically or eliminated by a variety of methods.

Excision Surgery: In this procedure, the endometrial lesion and its surrounding tissue are taken out. Because it eliminates the lesion completely, this approach is recommended as it lowers the chance of recurrence and offers more thorough pain relief.

When endometriosis affects vital structures like the bladder, diaphragm, or colon, excision surgery is advised instead of ablation since it is frequently more successful in treating moderate to severe cases of the condition.

Ablation Surgery: Endometrial lesions are destroyed on their surface using heat or a laser. Although this technique helps reduce pain, it may leave deeper, more invasive tissue behind and does not completely eradicate the lesion.

Because of this, ablation is less successful than excision and is typically reserved for situations that are milder or when prompt symptom alleviation is required.

Laparotomy: Open Surgery for Severe Cases A laparotomy is an open surgical technique in which the pelvic cavity is accessed by making a wider abdominal incision.

When minimally invasive methods are impractical and there is widespread disease in a case of severe endometriosis, this kind of surgery is usually reserved.

A laparotomy enables a more complete excision of endometrial tissue, particularly when adhesions have caused considerable organ damage or have fused organs together.

Hysterectomy: A Last Resort Procedure A hysterectomy entails the removal of the uterus along with the fallopian tubes (salpingectomy) and ovaries (oophorectomy) in certain situations.

Although a hysterectomy can ease pain associated with endometriosis, it is not a cure. Even after the uterus is removed, endometriosis may continue, especially if there is any endometrial tissue left in the pelvic cavity.

When all other options have failed and the woman does not want to have children in the future, a hysterectomy is typically seen as her last alternative.

Benefits and Risks of Surgical Options

Every surgical procedure carries risks and benefits, and these should be weighed carefully before deciding on a treatment plan.

Benefits of Surgery

When endometrial lesions, cysts, and adhesions are completely eliminated, surgery can significantly and occasionally immediately relieve pain.

By eliminating obstructions and reestablishing normal anatomy, surgery can increase a woman's chances of becoming pregnant if she has endometriosis-related infertility.

Following surgery, many patients report dramatic improvements in their quality of life, including less pain, more mobility, and improved general well being.

Risks of Surgery

Even with surgery, endometriosis can return, particularly if endometrial tissue is left behind or if ablation methods are employed rather than excision.

Possible side effects include bleeding, infection, damage to the bladder or intestines, and the development of adhesions, which are scar tissue formations that can hurt or clog the gut.

Fertility can be impacted by certain procedures (hysterectomy, for example), and adhesions from conservative surgery can occasionally damage reproductive organs.

Chapter Nine

Adolescent Endometriosis

Although endometriosis is frequently associated with adult women, it can start much earlier, even in youth. Living with endometriosis can be extremely difficult and isolating for young people, especially teens.

There are times when the symptoms are written off as "normal" menstrual discomfort, which delays identification and treatment. Teens suffering from endometriosis may encounter symptoms that are misinterpreted or disregarded by caregivers, educators, and medical professionals.

It is critical to understand that extreme menstruation pain in teenagers is not "normal" and shouldn't be written off as a natural aspect of growing up.

Teens suffering from endometriosis may report periods that hurt far more than regular menstrual pains. This pain might interfere with everyday activities, school attendance, and social contacts. It usually begins prior to menstruation and lasts the entire month.

Contrary to regular period pain, endometriosis-related pain might last all month long rather than just throughout the menstrual cycle. A young person's quality of life may be significantly impacted by this chronic pain, which can cause severe agony in the lower abdomen, back, and even legs.

Gastrointestinal problems in adolescents might include diarrhea, constipation, bloating, and nausea, particularly during their menstrual cycle. Delaying a correct diagnosis, these symptoms are frequently misdiagnosed as other illnesses, such as irritable bowel syndrome (IBS).

When participating in physical activities like sports or exercise, some teenagers with endometriosis experience pain that may be misinterpreted as a strain or injury to their muscles.

Anemia and exhaustion may result from heavy and extended monthly bleeding, which is another sign. Teenagers who are menstruating may need to replace their tampons or pads regularly and may have big clots of blood.

Challenges of Adolescent Diagnosis

Adolescent endometriosis diagnosis brings special difficulties. Teenage endometriosis symptoms are frequently disregarded or mistakenly linked to other illnesses because of the misconception that the disease typically affects older women.

Many teenagers are advised they are just being too sensitive or that their discomfort is a typical aspect of menstruation. When others close to them disregard their suffering, it can cause them to feel frustrated, alone, and powerless.

The symptoms of endometriosis might mimic those of other common adolescent illnesses, such as IBS, pelvic inflammatory disease (PID), or urinary tract infections (UTIs), which can result in incorrect diagnosis and treatment.

Both the general population and health care professionals are generally ignorant about endometriosis in teens. Many young people may have to wait years for a thorough diagnosis and appropriate care as a result, which can cause a major delay in diagnosis.

Adolescent Therapy

Teens with endometriosis should receive tailored treatment that takes into account their goal for future fertility, the severity of their symptoms, and the influence on their quality of life.

Hormonal medications, such as progestins, birth control tablets, or gonadotropin-releasing hormone (GnRH) agonists, are frequently used as the first line of treatment for teenagers in order to suppress the menstrual cycle and manage pain.

Pain and inflammation can also be reduced with the use of non-steroidal anti-inflammatory medications (NSAIDs).

A laparoscopy could be advised if medical therapy is not working or if endometriosis is suspected but not proven.

The endometrial lesions are removed or destroyed with this minimally invasive surgery, which enables identification and therapy. Nonetheless, adolescents undergoing surgery are advised to proceed cautiously, given the possible hazards and the significance of maintaining fertility.

Promoting a healthy lifestyle that includes regular exercise, a balanced diet, and stress reduction methods can help control symptoms and enhance general well being.

Teenagers dealing with endometriosis may benefit from emotional support and coping skills training offered by support groups and counseling.

Chapter Ten

Menopause and Endometriosis

Although endometriosis is frequently linked to women who are fertile, it can also develop, worsen, or even start during menopause.

Menopausal endometriosis patients suffer different symptoms and difficulties from their earlier years of the disease, necessitating a different approach to diagnosis and treatment.

The menstrual cycle's termination, or menopause, is commonly associated with a drop in estrogen levels. Many people with endometriosis think that their symptoms should go better after menopause because the ailment is thought to be estrogen-dependent. This isn't always the case, though.

Some people may experience endometriosis symptoms long after menopause. This may be caused by endometrial tissue that is still in the body and still causes discomfort and inflammation, especially in women who have had hormone replacement treatment (HRT) or who have elevated amounts of estrogen in their bloodstream by nature.

Rarely, endometriosis may be discovered for the first time during or following menopause. This may be connected to cases that were undetected or asymptomatic in the past, or it may be brought on by menopausal surgery or hormonal changes.

Hormone Replacement Therapy (HRT)

Hot flashes, nocturnal sweats, and dry vagina are among the menopausal symptoms that are frequently treated with hormone replacement therapy. HRT, however, presents particular difficulties for women who have a history of endometriosis.

Estrogen and Symptom Recurrence: Hormone replacement therapy (HRT), especially estrogen-only therapy, has the potential to accelerate the growth of leftover endometrial tissue, which could result in a relapse of endometriosis symptoms.

Women who have a history of endometriosis should talk to their doctor about the advantages and disadvantages of hormone replacement therapy (HRT), and if necessary, they should also investigate other options.

Combination HRT: By using progesterone and estrogen therapy together, some of the hazards related to estrogen-only HRT may be reduced. Progesterone may lessen the chance of endometrial tissue formation by balancing the effects of estrogen.

Non-Hormonal treatments: Non-hormonal treatments, such as dietary modifications, lifestyle changes, and medication, can assist control menopausal symptoms without raising the risk of recurrence of endometriosis in individuals who cannot or do not want to use HRT.

Considerations for Postmenopausal Women

Postmenopausal women who have endometriosis may have particular health consequences that need for cautious management and observation.

Risk of Ovarian Cancer: Research indicates that women who have endometriosis, particularly those who are postmenopausal, may be at slightly higher risk of developing ovarian cancer.

It's critical to keep an eye out for signs including bloating, pelvic pain, and adjustments to bowel or bladder habits. You should also talk to a health care professional about any worries you may have.

Adhesions and Scarring: Endometriosis-related adhesions and scarring can cause pain and discomfort long beyond menopause. Adhesions can cause intestinal blockage or persistent pelvic pain, which calls for continuing care and, in certain situations, surgery.

Osteoporosis and Bone Health: Women with endometriosis may be more susceptible to osteoporosis, especially if they have undergone long-term hormone suppression medication or have had their ovaries removed (oophorectomy).

Maintaining bone health requires routine bone density examinations as well as preventive interventions like vitamin D and calcium supplementation and weight-bearing exercise.

Symptoms After Menopause

A customized strategy is needed to manage endometriosis symptoms after menopause, taking into account the ongoing nature of the symptoms as well as the overall health requirements of older women.

For endometriosis-afflicted postmenopausal women, managing chronic pain is still a top issue. NSAIDs, physical therapy, acupuncture, and mindfulness-based stress reduction methods are among the available options.

Comprehensive care can be provided through a multidisciplinary approach comprising physical therapists, mental health doctors, and pain specialists.

Surgery might be required for certain women in order to treat chronic pain or other issues including intestinal obstruction. Depending on the extent of the disease and general health, surgical options range from less intrusive treatments to remove endometriotic lesions or adhesions to more involved procedures.

Keeping up a healthy lifestyle can aid with symptom management and well being enhancement. Exercise on a regular basis, a healthy diet full of foods high in anti-inflammatory foods, and stress reduction methods can all help to lower inflammation, elevate mood, and improve quality of life.

Healthy Aging with Endometriosis

Endometriosis-related aging poses special difficulties, but with the correct techniques, women can successfully control their symptoms and preserve a high quality of life.

Managing comorbidities, keeping an eye on any changes in symptoms, and maintaining general health all depend on routine visits to health care professionals.

Stressing a balanced diet, consistent exercise, and mental health techniques can enhance one's physical and mental well-being by fostering a sense of control and well being.

Appendix A: Glossary of Terms

This glossary provides definitions of key terms used throughout the book, helping you better understand the language used by health care professionals.

Ablation: *A surgical procedure that destroys endometrial lesions using heat or laser.*

Adhesions: *Bands of scar tissue that can form between organs and tissues, often causing pain or complications.*

Dysmenorrhea: *Painful menstrual periods, which can be severe and debilitating in endometriosis.*

Endometriomas: *A type of ovarian cyst formed from endometrial tissue, often filled with dark, thickened blood.*

Excision Surgery: *A surgical procedure that removes endometrial lesions and surrounding tissue.*

Laparoscopy: *A minimally invasive surgical procedure used to diagnose and treat endometriosis.*

Pelvic Inflammatory Disease (PID): *An infection of the female reproductive organs, which can mimic some symptoms of endometriosis.*

Retrograde Menstruation: *A condition where menstrual blood flows backward into the pelvic cavity, potentially leading to endometriosis.*

Appendix B: Resources and Support Organizations

Endometriosis can be challenging, but you don't have to do it alone. This appendix lists resources and support organizations that provide information, support, and advocacy for those affected by endometriosis.

Endometriosis Association

Provides educational resources, support groups, and research funding to improve the lives of those affected by endometriosis.

Website: *www.endometriosisassn.org*

Endometriosis Foundation of America

Offers patient advocacy, awareness campaigns, and research initiatives focused on endometriosis.

Website: *www.endofound.org*

Center for Endometriosis Care

Specializes in the comprehensive care and treatment of endometriosis, including minimally invasive surgery.

Website: *www.centerforendo.com*

The American College of Obstetricians and Gynecologists (ACOG)

Provides guidelines, educational materials, and resources for patients and health care providers.

Website: *www.acog.org*

Pelvic Pain Support Network

Focuses on providing support and information to individuals suffering from chronic pelvic pain, including endometriosis.

Website: *www.pelvicpain.org.uk*

The End

9 798344 729688